I0791083

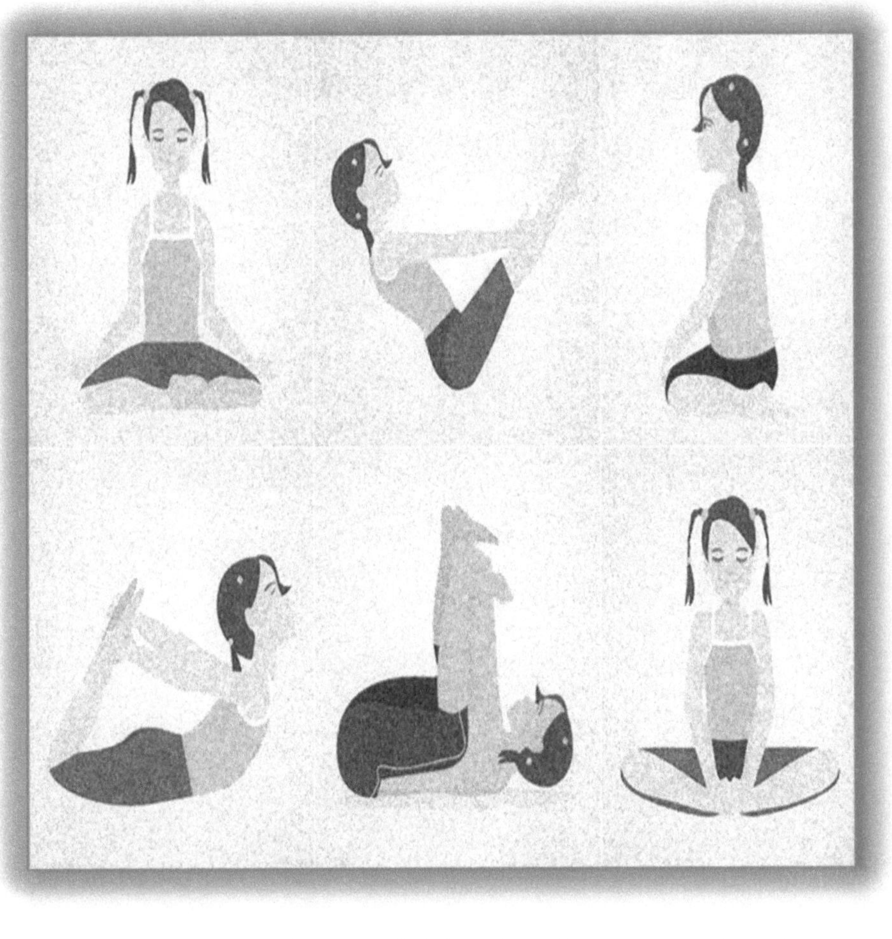

THE BEST YOGA POSES FOR KIDS

WRITTEN BY DEBRA STEPHENS

TABLE OF CONTENT

CHAPTER ONE:

WHAT IS YOGA?

Yoga can be seen as a psyche and body practice with
a 5,000-year history in the old Indian way of thinking.
Different styles of yoga join physical stances,
breathing procedures, and contemplation, or
unwinding.

Research expresses that yoga activities may assist
youngsters with adapting to pressure and have
equalization throughout everyday life and emotional
wellness. A kid doesn't require yoga abilities to begin
rehearsing it. They simply need to begin, and yoga
will turn into a method for their life. It keeps them
dynamic, balances their body, psyche, and soul, and
encourages them to center around their life.

This book causes you to acquaint yoga with your
youngsters, as we inform you concerning the
advantages of yoga for children and offer directions
for some straightforward yoga asanas (yoga presents)
in the first place.

CHAPTER TWO:

INTRODUCTION: WHAT ARE THE BENEFITS OF YOGA FOR KIDS?

Yoga is a way of thinking that shows the capacity to join the physical, otherworldly, and passionate parts of an individual and causes them to arrive at a condition of inward harmony and care.

It is a smart thought to begin instructing yoga to kids at an early age, as it isn't just useful to their physical development but in addition to their emotion and by and large prosperity in both health and life. It likewise causes youngsters to create relational connections, stress management, and care, abilities that may be valuable in their adulthood.

Yoga might be useful while managing a few physical and enthusiastic issues. It could be utilized as an apparatus to get a parity life. Here are a portion of the conceivable medical advantages of yoga:

- Improves body equalization, quality, and vigorous limit

- Help decrease incessant torment, for example, muscle torment

- Enhances the nature of rest

- Can lessen the arrival of stress hormones like cortisone, and, in this way, is successful in diminishing pressure, uneasiness, and weakness

- Works on the kid's study hall conduct, center, and scholarly execution

- Improves personal satisfaction by bringing enthusiastic parity, since yoga is a non-focused movement

- Helps kids improve strength, state of mind, and self-guideline aptitudes

- Six long periods of yoga, including reflection, asanas, and pranayama (breathing activities), have appeared to diminish body weight, improve endocrine capacities and memory

Yoga has endless advantages to offer. Let your child start with the essential postures and understand the magnificence of this training. There are various styles of yoga, including body stances, breathing activities, and reflection. In this way, while showing yoga for kids, you may think about concentrating on the development and on the best way to make it fascinating for them at first. When you can get them intrigued, consider including breathing and contemplation.

You ought to likewise disclose to your kid that they could receive the rewards of yoga after some time, and to accomplish this, they have to rehearse it routinely.

In any case, here are a couple of simple yoga presents you can take a stab at showing your youngsters.

CHAPTER THREE:

15 SPECIAL AND HIGHLY EFFECTIVE YOGA POSES FOR KIDS

Yoga doesn't require a gigantic place or expand hardware. It tends to be acted in the nursery, home, or at school, with only a yoga tangle.

Here are some yoga models for kids; they are simple, snappy, and ok for ordinary practice.

1. Bridge Pose Also Called – Setu Banda Sarvangasana:

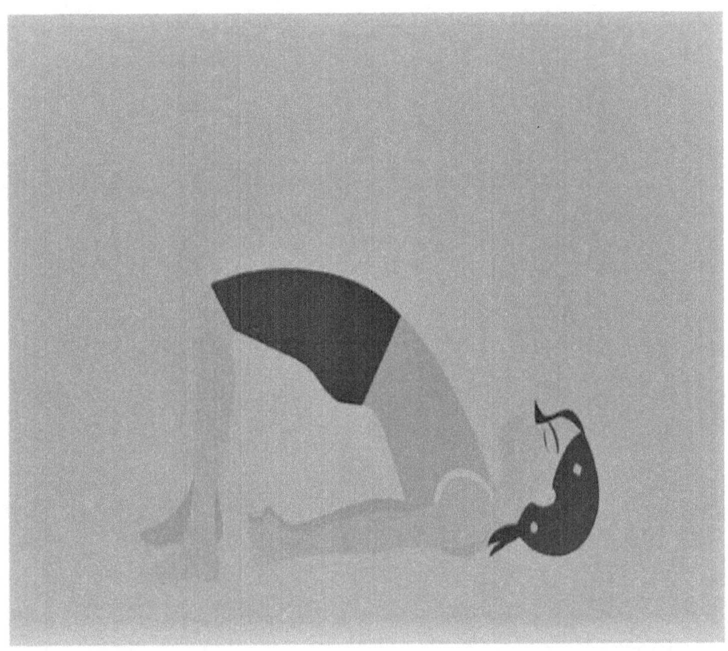

This reviving backbend gives a decent stretch to the spine and thighs.

Step by step instructions to do:

1.   Lie on the back.

2.   Bend the knees a little and keep the feet level on the floor, hip-width separated.

3.   The knees and lower legs must be in a straight line.

4.   Place the arms in a resting position close to the body, with the palms downwards.

5.   Take a full breath and lift the lower, center, and upper back off the floor.

6.   Balance the body such that the arms, shoulders, and feet bolster the body weight.

7.   Keep the backside tight.

8.   Have the fingers interweaved, and hands pushed to the ground to help lift the middle higher.

9.   Let your youngster hold this stance for whatever length of time that they are agreeable and inhale gradually while they are in the posture.

10.   Exhale and discharge.

Potential advantages: Stretches and opens the shoulders, thighs, hips, and chest partition; fortifies the back and hamstrings; expands the adaptability of the spine

Alert: If your child faces trouble in making the pelvis lift from the floor, slide a tough reinforce under their sacrum to rest their pelvis. In the event of any neck or shoulder torment, take help from an expert to sharpen the means.

2. Tree Pose Also Called – Vrksasana:

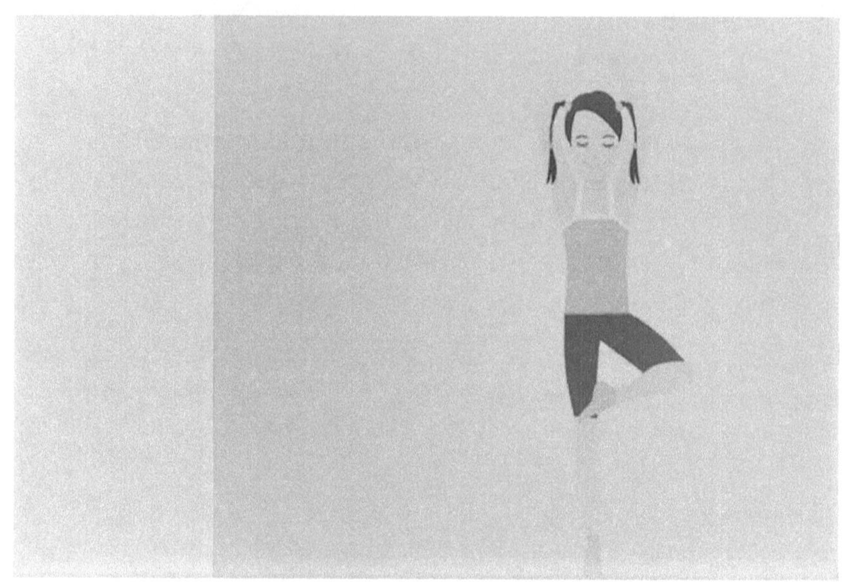

Vrksasana shows your child the finesse of a tree, standing tall and looking after equalization.

Step by step instructions to do:

1.   Begin the stance with the mountain present, wherein the legs are straight, hands along the edges, back straight, and thigh muscles firm.

2.   Lift the correct foot with the knee out.

3.	Place the correct foot on the left internal thigh in a position where it feels great.

4.	Press the hands together over the head.

5.	Gaze at a point around five feet away.

6.	Hold the situation for 30 seconds to a moment.

7.	Return the hands to the chest and afterward bring down the correct leg.

8.	Repeat it on the left leg.

Potential advantages: Improves equalization and focus; fortifies the thigh muscles, calves, and lower legs while extending the legs and the chest

Alert: If your child gets flimsy first and foremost while attempting to hold their stance, you may make them remain with their back against a divider.

2. Cobra Pose Also Called – Bhujangasana:

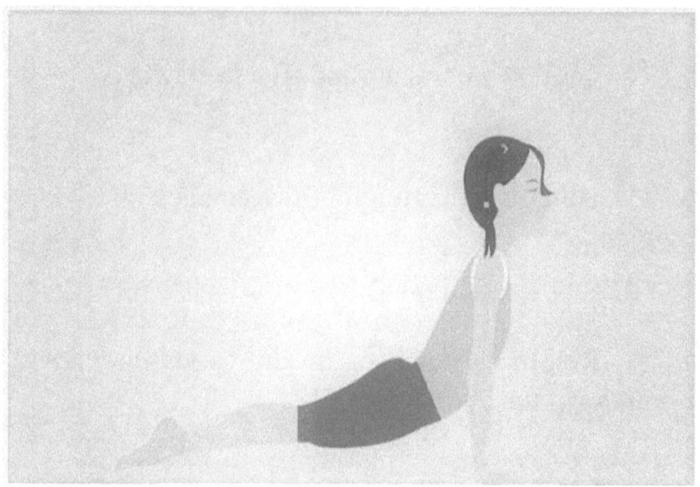

The stretch may advance a tough back, abs, and quality.

The most effective method to do:

1.   Lie face down with the tips of the feet level on the floor and palms on either side of the body.

2.   Pull the shoulders marginally back towards the spine.

3.   Engage the guts all through the activity as it holds the lower back secured.

4.   Lift the body into a cobra present while keeping the jaw up. Utilize the hands for help, however without putting pointless weight.

5.   Hold the stance for 15 to 30 seconds, before delicately discharging the body to the floor. This is a decent, morning yoga present for children to rehearse day by day.

Potential advantages: Strengthens the spine; extends the chest, shoulders, stomach area, and hindquarters; animates the stomach organs and discharges weariness and stress; may be useful for overseeing breathing issues like asthma.

Alert: Ask your child to curve the back as much as the body can take. Each youngster has distinctive adaptability, so let them move slowly.

3. Cat Pose Also Called – Marjaryasana:

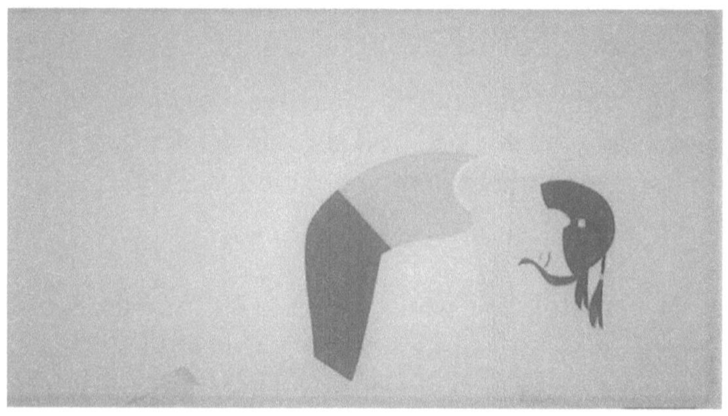

The feline posture is a delicate plying for the back and center.

The most effective method to do:

1.   Take a tabletop position utilizing the hands and knees.

2.   Your knees ought to be straightforwardly beneath the hips, and toes twisted.

3.   The wrists, elbows, and shoulders ought to be straight and opposite to the floor.

4.   Center your head in an unbiased situation with eyes taking a gander at the floor.

5.   With an exhalation, curve the spine up towards the roof.

6.   Release your head towards the floor without driving your jawline towards the chest.

7.   Come back to the underlying tabletop position while breathing in gradually.

Potential advantages: Relaxes and stretches the spine, neck, middle, and the organs of the stomach area

Alert: If your child faces trouble while adjusting their upper back, lay a hand above and between the shoulder bones for help.

5. Bow Pose Also Called – Dhanurasana:

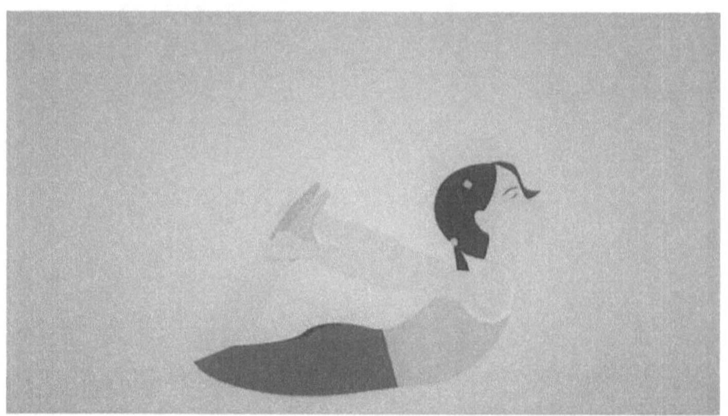

Twist the back like a bow and open the chest and shoulders with the bow present.

Step by step instructions to do:

1.   Lie level on your stomach, keeping your arms extended at the edges of your body and head laying delicately on the tangle.

2.   Inhale and twist your knees bringing your feet towards your hips.

3.	Grasp your lower legs utilizing both your hands.

4.	Lift your shoulders, middle, legs, and hips off the floor while looking straight ahead.

5.	Hold your stance for four to five breaths, at that point bring down your knees and discharge your feet.

6.	Rest on your stomach.

Potential advantages: Stretches and fortifies the back, shoulders, chest, and legs; carries adaptability to hip flexor work, and directs the stomach related framework

Alert: The bow present includes a lot of extending, so if your youngster feels overwhelming in the lower back, keep the stance lower until it is agreeable to extend. Help them in holding the lower legs in stage 3 and lifting the body in stage 4.

6. Frog Pose Also Called – Mandukasana:

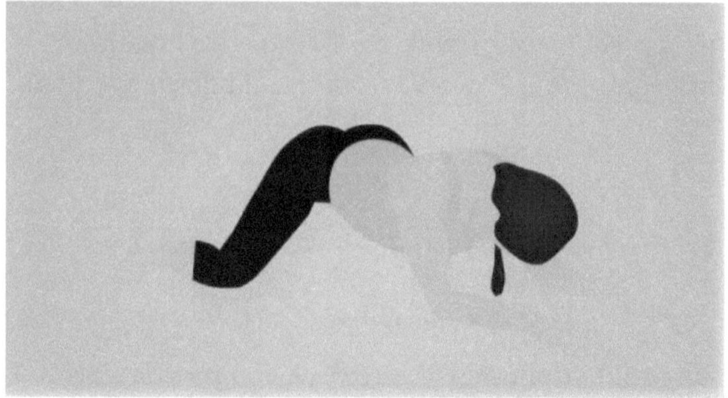

This posture may help in soothing sprains or back agonies.

The most effective method to do:

1.   Start by going on the floor with your hands and knees on the floor.

2.   Position your knees a couple of inches separated and place your feet directly behind your knees.

3.   Place your palms directly under your shoulders with your fingers looking ahead.

4.   Look downwards and center at a point between your hands.

5.   Now, push your tailbone towards the back. This will extend your spine. This position is commonly known as the table position.

6.   Slowly move your knees outwards to your sides. At that point adjust your lower legs and feet to your knees in a straight line.

7.   Start to slide downwards while keeping the palms level against the floor.

8.   Exhale and continue pushing your hips in reverse until a stretch is felt.

9.   Now, hold this situation for three to five breaths.

10.   Come back to the table position once more.

Potential advantages: Stretches the hips, thighs, and spine

Alert: If it harms your kid under the knees or the elbows, place a collapsed cover to offer help and quality. Let them not extend past their solace level.

7. Easy Pose - Sukhasana:

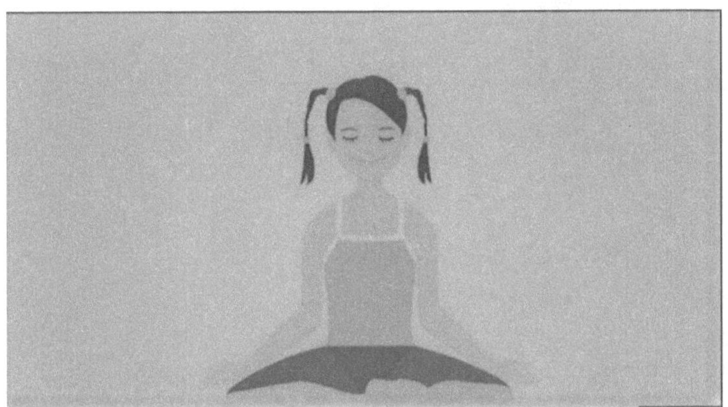

This is the easiest of all poses that the kid can attempt.

The most effective method to do:

1.   Sit upstanding with legs crossed.

2.   Rest your hands on your knees with your palms looking up.

3.   Evenly parity the weight over the sit bones.

4.	Keep your head, neck, and spine adjusted from the beginning.

5.	Elongate your spine yet without stiffing your neck.

6.	Your feet and thighs ought to be loose.

7.	Retain this stance for a moment.

8.	Release and change the leg over leg position.

Advantages: Good for the back, thighs, and hips; gives a stretch to the knees and feet; and aides in nullifying uneasiness and stress.

Alert: If your child's hips are tight and they are thinking that it's hard to sit level, prop them up with a collapsed cover or firm pad under the hips.

8. Butterfly Pose Also Called – Baddha Konasana:

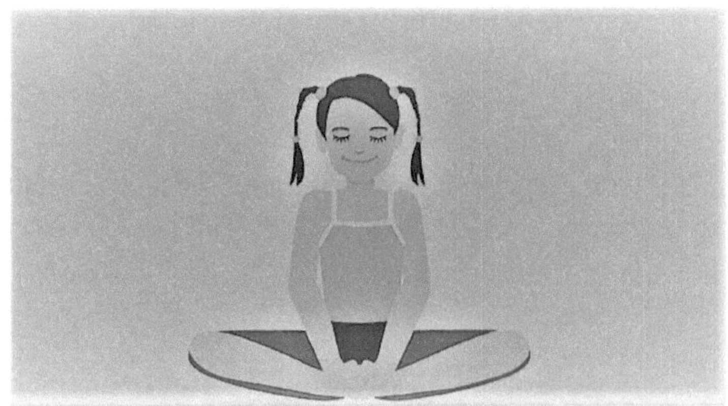

A represent that makes your child vacillate like a smooth butterfly, this is accepted to offer some significant advantages.

Step by step instructions to do:

1.   Sit with your spine upstanding and legs spread out straight.

2.   Fold the legs with the goal that your feet are contacting one another. Hold them with the hands.

3.   While breathing out, tenderly move the thighs and knees in a descending movement.

4.   Then beginning fluttering the advantages and down, similar to the wings of a butterfly.

5.   The fluttering ought to be moderate at first and afterward get a move on. Breathing ought to be at an ordinary pace.

6.   Slow down bit by bit and afterward stop.

7.   Gently discharge the stance while breathing out.

Potential advantages: Stretches the thighs, knees, and hips; directs the digestive tract and solid discharge; for young ladies, helps in simple and effortless feminine cycle.

Alert: If your child has a knee or crotch damage, hold a cover under the thighs to counteract agony or hurt.

9. Corpse Pose Also Called - Savasana:

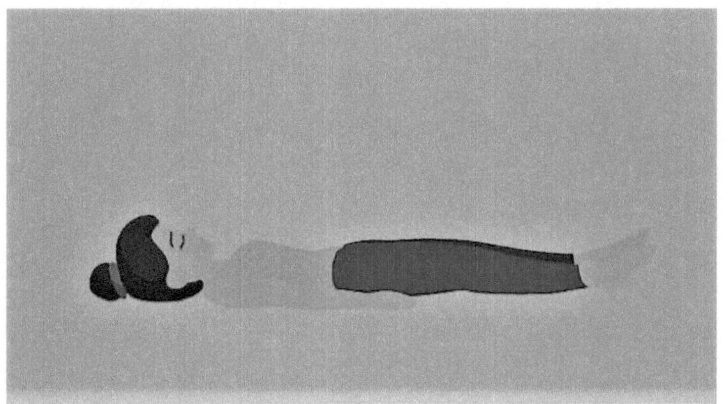

A represent that makes your child vacillate like a smooth butterfly, this is accepted to offer some significant advantages.

Step by step instructions to do:

1.   Sit with the spine upstanding and legs spread out straight.

2.   Fold the legs with the goal that the feet are contacting one another. Hold them with the hands.

3.   While breathing out, tenderly move the thighs and knees in a descending movement.

4.   Then beginning fluttering your advantages and down, similar to the wings of a butterfly.

5.   The fluttering ought to be moderate at first and afterward get a move on. Breathing ought to be at an ordinary pace.

6.   Slow down bit by bit and afterward stop.

7.   Gently discharge your stance while breathing out.

Potential advantages: Stretches the thighs, knees, and hips; directs the digestive tract and solid discharge; for young ladies, helps in simple and effortless feminine cycle.

Alert: If your child has a knee or crotch damage, hold a cover under the thighs to counteract agony or hurt.

10. Chair pose Also Called - Utkatasana:

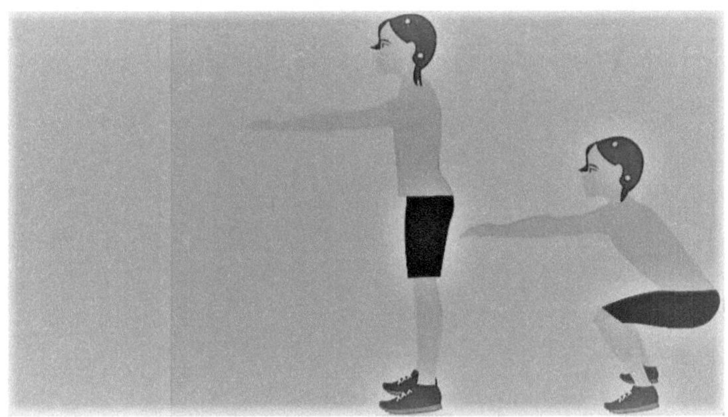

The seat post is an exercise for the legs, arms, and the heart, and is accepted to be one of the most productive yoga presents.

Instructions to do:

1.   Inhale and raise your arms over your head.

2.   Bend your knees forward while breathing out; your thighs ought to be parallel to the floor.

3.   While performing it, the knees will extend marginally ahead.

4.   Lift your arms and stretch them straight.

5.   Keep your tailbone down and your lower back long.

6.   Keep your breath consistent and simple all through.

7.   Keep your look forward.

8.   Retain this stance for whatever length of time that agreeable, however not over a moment.

Potential advantages: Works on the thigh muscles and lower legs; conditions the shoulders, hips, and the spine; controls the stomach related framework and heart working.

Alerts: If your youngster is encountering cerebral pains or a sleeping disorder, don't play out this asana.

11. Hero Pose also called – Virasana:

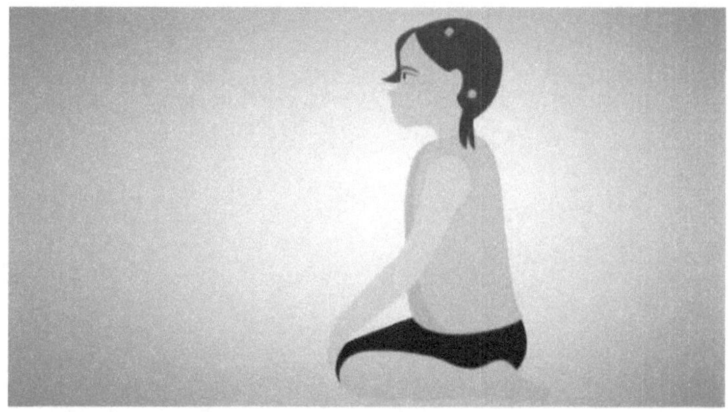

This posture may be the ointment for the exhausted legs of your children.

The most effective method to do:

1.	Sit with your knees together and your feet hip-width separated.

2.	Sit on your heels with your heels contacting your hips.

3.	Your hands should lay on your knees with your palms looking up.

4.   Straighten your spine and drop your shoulders down and a little towards the back.

5.   Relax your center while taking full breaths.

6.   Retain your stance for whatever length of time that it is agreeable.

Potential advantages: Stretches the spine, quadriceps, and shoulders; improves blood course and diminishes tiredness of legs; improves assimilation and stance.

Alert: If the hips don't lay serenely on the yoga tangle, utilize a yoga obstruct in the middle.

12. Boat Pose Also Called - Naukasana:

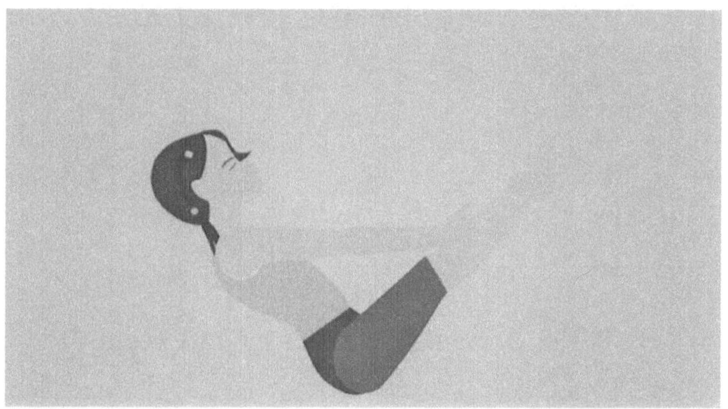

This adjusting yoga posture may help children to de-stretch and renew.

The most effective method to do:

1.   Lie down level with feet adjusted together and arms on the sides.

2.   Keep your arms and fingers outstretched toward your toes.

3.   Inhale and keeping in mind that breathing out, lifts your chest and feet off the ground, to frame an 'Angular' shape.

4.   This will assemble strain and stretch in your center.

5.   The load of your body will exclusively lay on your hips.

6.   The eyes, hands, and toes ought to adjust straight.

7.   Hold your breath and hold your stance for a couple of moments.

8.   Exhale gradually while bringing your body down to the impartial position. What's more, unwind.

Potential advantages: Strengthens the center, arm muscles, shoulders, and thighs; it is incredible for the liver and kidneys; lessens stoppage and reduces stomach related issues.

Alert: If your child experiences any incessant sickness or spinal string issues, evade the posture.

13. Mountain Pose Also Called - Tadasana:

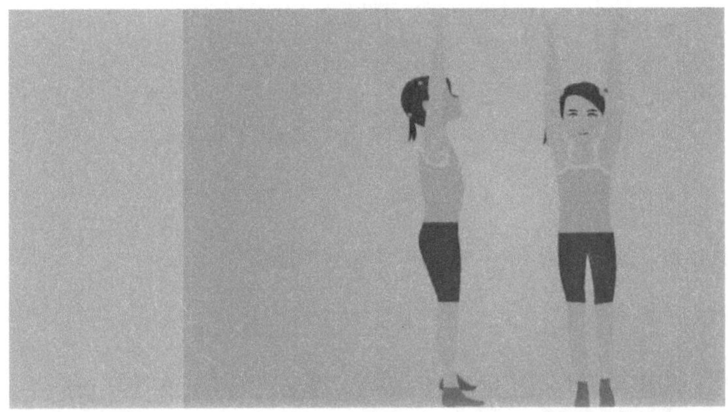

This is a primary posture for all the standing asanas and could be a quiet down yoga present for youngsters.

The most effective method to do:

1.   Stand straight and tall.

2.   Spread your legs a couple of inches separated and spread your toes.

3.   Keep your arms close by your body.

4.   Your shoulders must be loose and not hardened.

5.   Raise your arms over your head.

6.   Hold your stance and inhale gradually.

7.   Retain as long as agreeable.

Potential advantages: Improves act, reinforces the thighs, legs, and lower legs; firms the belly and hips; improves rest

Alert: No alerts to development.

14. Happy Baby Pose Also Called – Ananda Balasana:

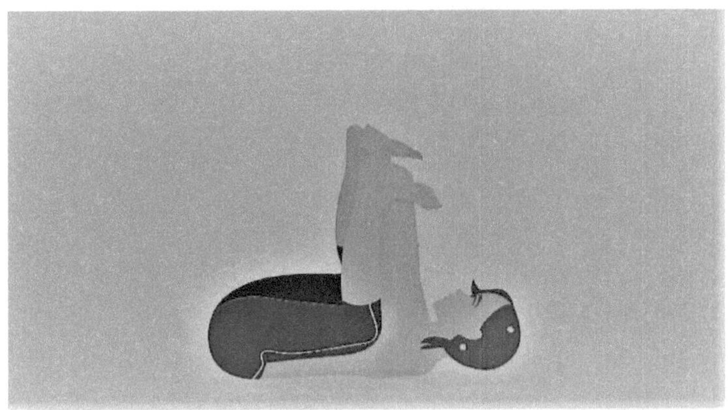

This asana may help loosen up your back joints.

The most effective method to do:

1.   Lie on your back with your knees attracted towards your chest.

2.   Hold your feet with hands. Guarantee that your arms are before your middle.

3.   Draw your shoulders to the back.

4.   Slightly stretch your arms and feet.

5.   Draw your knees wide separated, as much as agreeable.

6.   Elongate the drop down to the ground while contacting the tip of the tailbone.

7.   Retain the situation for a moment or less, and afterward discharge.

Potential advantages: Stretches and opens the hips, thighs and inward crotch; extends the spine; reinforces the arms and shoulders

Alert: If your child has any knee or lower leg damage, check with a specialist before playing out this posture.

15. Lion Pose Also Called - Simhasana:

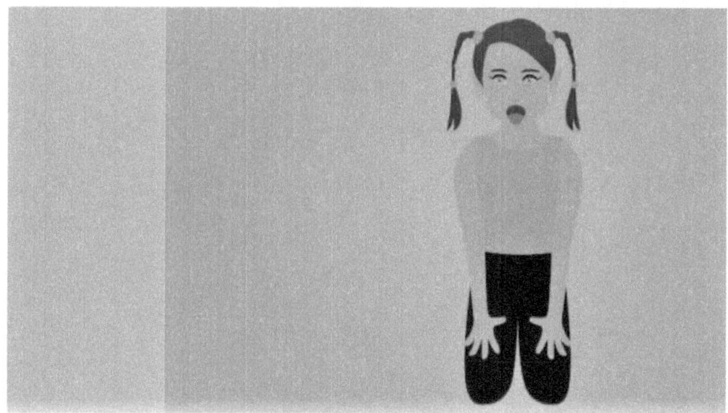

Might help your youngster de-worry with this creature asana; have them thunder and appreciate.

The most effective method to do:

1.   Sit with your hips on your heels.

2.   Rest your palms on your knees.

3.   Start breathing in from the nose, and keeping in mind that you're on it, stick your tongue out.

4.   Keep your eyes all the way open, breathe out through your mouth, and make a sound of a thundering lion (Haaa).

5.   Many yoga schools recommend that you either accumulate taking a gander at the tip of the nose or in the eyebrows.

Potential advantages: An incredible yoga stretch for the lungs, throat, and the respiratory tract; controls the working of the tonsils and the invulnerable framework; diminishes pressure, outrage, and nervousness; reasonable for a hyperactive kid.

Alert: Do not rehash this for in excess of multiple times.

An everyday schedule of yoga movement will make your kid increasingly taught and concentrated on their action and invigorates them the to confront pressure. Start with a couple of yoga stances to rehearse at first, and afterward you can have them attempt more as they become acclimated to the training.

www.ingramcontent.com/pod-product-compliance
Lightning Source LLC
Chambersburg PA
CBHW051132250726
48655CB00007B/3018